The Effectiveness of Continuing Professional Development

KW-126-512

CONTENTS

DEVELOPMENT:

A report for the Chief Medical Officer's review of continuing professional development in practice.

Janet Grant and Frances Stanton

The Joint Centre for Education in Medicine,
London

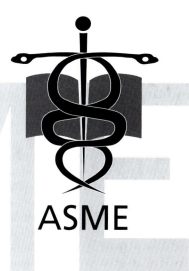

ASME

ASME Office
12 Queen Street
Edinburgh
EH2 1JE

No part of this book may be copied or reproduced without permission.

First published by
Joint Centre for Education in Medicine,
33 Millman Street, London, WC1N 3EJ, UK

Republished by ASME January 2000

ISBN: 0904473260

Further copies of this and other ASME medical education booklets are available from the ASME office. For a price list and order form contact:

Telephone 0131 225 9111
Fax 0131 225 9444
Email: info@asme.org.uk
http://www.asme.org.uk

When citing this book, use the following notation:

Grant J and Stanton F
ASME Occasional Publication
The Effectiveness of Continuing Professional Development: A report for the Chief Medical Officer's review of continuing professional development in practice.
Association for the Study of Medical Education, Edinburgh, 1999.

Correspondence to : Professor Janet Grant, 27 Church Street, Hampton, Middlesex, TW12 2EB, UK.

INTRODUCTION

This report addresses the literature and issues surrounding evidence and subsequent policy in relation to the effectiveness of continuing professional development activities. The need for, and challenges of, an evidential basis of effectiveness, and justification for subsequent strategic decisions, are addressed. The report will show that the evidence is often weak and inconclusive. Nonetheless, there are some highly significant messages which indicate positive ways ahead. These messages are substantial enough to pool together and offer a foundation for subsequent strategy.

The main message to emerge is that the key to lifelong, effective learning is not to be found in advice about how to learn but rather in how to *manage* the learning process. The finding that, for CPD, that process might best be managed in the context of practice might also imply that the effective management of learning might be different at different stages of undergraduate, postgraduate and continuing education.

Continuing professional development (CPD) is concerned with the acquisition, enhancement and maintenance of knowledge, skills and attitudes by professional practitioners, and its broad aims are to enhance professionals' performance and optimise the outcomes of their practice[1,2]. In relation to medicine therefore it can be described as:

....promoting high quality and up-to-date patient care by ensuring that all clinicians have the learning opportunities to maintain and improve their competence to practice[3].

The provision of formal CPD activities in the form of educational meetings has increased dramatically over the past 20 years or so, both in medicine and across a wide variety of other professions. Corresponding increases have been seen in the resources expended in connection with its provision[4] and in the amount of research which it has generated[5]. These increases have been prompted and encouraged by changes both in the content and contexts of modern professions[1] and in Government policy [such as, for example, the 'New Contracts' (1989) and the three 1996 White Papers concerned with the operation of the NHS in general (one paper) and of primary care in particular (two papers)].

The purpose of this paper is to review the recent literature in this area[1] to discover the relative effectiveness of different CPD activities, in terms of the achievement of the aims of CPD, and to isolate those strategies and features which have been shown to promote effectiveness. To place these findings in context, however, a brief overview will first be presented of the nature and prevalence of CPD, its aims and functions, and the educational approaches adopted in its provision. Influences on the extent and type of CPD programmes offered and on participation in such programmes will also be mentioned, and the numerous and complex methodological issues relevant to the study of the effectiveness of CPD will be discussed.

Information has been drawn primarily from health care and educational literature as well as that specifically related to medicine. Findings will be discussed both in general terms and with particular reference to outcomes relevant to the medical and related professions. It has not proved either necessary or appropriate for all the papers in the reference list to be cited individually in the body of this review, but all have been drawn on to inform what has been written.

CONTINUING PROFESSIONAL DEVELOPMENT IN CONTEXT

2.1 The nature and prevalence of CPD

There is general agreement across the literature about the broad definition and aims of CPD given above. At more specific levels, however, agreement is less common and a degree of confusion about the exact nature of CPD is apparent. A large part of this confusion arises from, and is evident in, the use of terminology: CPD developed out of the earlier concepts of continuing professional education (CPE) and continuing medical education (CME). The terms 'education' and 'development' do not refer to exactly the same thing, but the distinction between them is not always reflected in the way they are used, either in the literature or in practice. This has partly resulted from the fact that changes in both the conceptualisation and the practice of ongoing professional learning took place before a new term was adopted to take account of the new concepts and practices.

Formal CME provision traditionally emphasised teacher-based, didactic approaches, but such approaches have recently been criticised and the need for more learner-led approaches to be included in CPD programmes has become apparent[6,7]. Awareness has also increased of the existing prevalence of self-directed, opportunistic and informal learning among professionals and of the role this has to play in their ongoing development: Gear et al.[8], for example, propose that most 'continuous learning' is likely to be initiated, organised, controlled and evaluated by the individual, and that formal inputs play only a supporting role. However, this predeliction for self-direction in learning does not in any way imply that doctors do not like to have their learning needs met by formal educational meetings. Indeed, a recent survey of general practitioners in their first 3 years of practice shows that (a) they do identify learning needs from their own practice and (b) they choose to meet these needs by short, formal educational meetings[9].

In medicine the inadequacy of the existing terms has been further highlighted by the increasing need for coverage of topics not normally forming part of traditional specialist education, such as management and communication skills training, teamwork and ethics[3]. CPD, as a term, reflects all these changes in the provision and perception of professionals' ongoing learning, and the practice of CPD within medicine is a development and extension of CPE and CME[2]. A description of CPD which reflects these changes is given by Todd (p. 5[10]) who suggests that CPD:

....makes no preconceptions about whether people learn or are taught, or about the formality of learning activities. People can develop themselves; others can also help them develop; the important thing is that professional development occurs.

While CPD is a very new term, however, CPE and CME were themselves relatively new areas of interest. Although the first reported CME course took place in 1935 and there were medical societies, associations and journals which performed a CME function in the 19th Century[11], CME was not discussed as a coherent body of literature until Sheperd's 1960 review[12] and the first reported conference dedicated to CME did not take place until as late as 1986[13]. The current prevalence of achievement of credit points for CPD both across professions and within medicine is, however, not entirely surprising given the governmental prescription that continuing education and training should be provided which meet the needs of multidisciplinary health care teams and their practices, and its stated ambition for '....a high quality, integrated health service which responds to the health needs of individual patients sensitively and cost effectively'[14] (p. 817). As Sackin[15] (p. 2) points out, with respect to general practice: '...if any practices have so far avoided "in-house" education, they can hardly get away without it now'!

In defining CME/CPD, we should also define strategies which can generate changes in practice, but which are not primarily educational, and therefore are largely excluded from this review. For example, Allery et al.[16] indicate that organisational factors are effective in inducing change. Other strategies of managing change will also have effect[17]. Computing may help improve clinician performance[18]. The classification of clinical guidelines is more problematic. They may be regarded as an assistance to practitioner decisions about appropriate care but might also be most effective when introduced through a specific educational programme, backed up by instrumental reminders to the clinician at the time of consultation[19]. This review will focus on educational interventions per se but will also address such associated contextual factors.

2.2 The aims and functions of CPD

2.2.1 Types of CPD model
Nowlem[20] has outlined three types of model on which CME programmes might be based, and the aims each typically sets out to achieve.

'Update models' underpin those programmes which aim simply to communicate or disseminate information. While this is a valid aim, there is a danger with this type of model that the acquisition of information may not be translated into improvements in practice[21,22].

'Competence models' aim to ensure that at least minimum standards for knowledge, skills and attitudes are attained. Programmes based on this type of model may be sufficient to provoke alterations of practice, but they do not necessarily address the issue of whether such alterations lead to optimised patient care outcomes.

'Performance models' (which were just beginning to gain prominence at the time at which he was writing) aim not only to help doctors overcome barriers to successful changes in practice, but also to help them resolve clinical concerns. In the medical field therefore some emphasis would be placed on health care outcomes.

Harden & Laidlaw[23] offer an approach to CPD which also recognises its integration with practice and places this in the wider context of the design of learning. Their CRISIS criteria emphasise the following points:

- *Convenience.* Makes voluntary participation easy.
- *Relevance.* Reflects the user's day-to-day role in medical practice.
- *Individualisation.* Allows learners a say in what is learnt and to adapt the programme to their own needs.
- *Self-assessment.* Encourages doctors to evaluate their understanding of the subject and to remedy any gaps identified.
- *Interest.* Gains attention and encourages learners to participate in the programme.
- *Speculation.* Recognises controversial and grey areas in medicine.
- *Systematic.* Offers a planned programme, with coverage of a whole subject or an identified part of it.

2.2.2 Aims
Despite the increasing prominence of performance models since the late 1980s, many programmes and authors still do not focus explicitly on aiming to change the outcomes of practice, possibly because they assume that these ought to follow automatically from changes in practice itself. Allery et al.[16], for example, give changes in doctors' behaviour as one of the important aims of CPD in medicine, while Chambers[7] favours the active fostering of practical competence. Wilbur[13], in his report of the first dedicated CME conference, records a proposal for CME to occur at, and be relevant to, the workplace, and for programmes to be aimed directly at deficiencies in practice, so that knowledge

acquired would be directly relevant to areas of need and therefore more likely to be applied to practice. Abernethy[21], on the other hand, makes direct reference to patient outcomes, stating that:

The whole purpose of continuing medical education is to improve the performance of the doctor in his practice and thus improve the care that patients receive.(p. 847)

Similarly, the Royal College of Obstetricians & Gynaecologists[2] designed their CME programme with the express purpose of encouraging trained specialist staff to update themselves regularly with respect to new knowledge, skills and procedures, to maintain the standards of clinical excellence needed for the optimal care of patients, and they argue that it is *in the public interest* for individual doctors to ensure their own sound professional development.

2.2.3 Functions

It would seem logical that perceptions of the functions of CPD would reflect its aims, and in some instances this is indeed the case. Parboosingh & Thivierge[25], for example, stress the increasing role of CME in the maintenance of professional competence. Less positively, but still relevant to the stated aims of CPD, Brennan's[26] review of CPE in four disciplines in Australia (the law, medicine, engineering, and teaching of mathematics and science) found varied perceptions of the importance and purpose of CPE. Not surprisingly, those unclear about the importance of CME were found to offer it only a limited purpose, but even when its importance was recognised, it was still not always viewed as having the potential to promote change in professional practice. In some cases, however, CPD is perceived to carry benefits additional to those arising from the achievement of its stated aims. For example, Branthwaite *et al.*[27] suggest that attendance at CME courses gives general practitioners (GPs) the following opportunities in addition to those for the acquisition of knowledge and the development and maintenance of high professional standards:

- maintenance of interests;
- encouragement of an ethos of keeping up-to-date;
- stimulation and motivation;
- provision of reassurance;
- provision of contact and comparison with other GPs;
- enhancement of group identity and confidence.

The issue of the confidence that others (patients, the public and managers) have in the doctor is another area in which CPD may serve as an enhancing factor[3]. The Royal Colleges of Physicians[28] also sees a more public benefit to widespread participation in CPD (p.iii).

Given the rapid advances in medical science, the greater expectations of an increasingly informed public and the growing tendency to apportion blame, it is inevitable that we must not only keep abreast of the latest developments, but also that we are seen to do so.

As well as having stated aims which are wholly worthwhile in their own right, CPD also has the potential to fulfil a greater role, both in terms of the development of the individual and of the impressions held of practitioners by others.

2.3 Educational approaches, learning and CPD

With increasing calls for the formal documentation and recognition of CPD within medicine, and with changes in specialist training meaning that hospital doctors begin CPD activities earlier than in the past[3], decisions about which activities and approaches to learning should be recognised as acceptable constituents of CPD are gaining in importance. As Gray[29] points out, a key question now is, how best can large numbers of doctors be encouraged and supported throughout a lifetime of development in professional practice.

The criticisms of the traditional approaches used in formal CME programmes have already been mentioned, and Moore's[30] is representative of the majority of these. He argues that the features of traditional CME:

- are lecture-dominated;
- are episodic and non-reinforcing;
- involve minimal collaboration between learners and providers;
- lack responsiveness to learner needs;
- place too much emphasis on the acquisition of credits;
- focus too heavily on course production.

In the light of these factors, the principles and features of adult learning are increasingly being brought into discussions of the nature and provision of CPD[13,22,25,31]. The following extract from Brookfield[32] (chapter 2) illustrates some of the key features of adult learning theory.

Adults learn throughout their lives....They exhibit diverse learning styles....and learn in different ways, at different times, for different purposes. As a rule, however, they like their learning activities to be problem centred and to be meaningful to their life situation, and they want the learning outcomes to have some immediacy of application. The past experience of adults affects their current learning, sometimes serving as an enhancement, sometimes as a hindrance. Effective learning is also linked to the adult's subscription to a self-concept of himself or herself as a learner. Finally, adults exhibit a tendency towards self-directedness in their learning.

Following Brookfield's view of adult learning, a number of authors propose that self-directed learning, based on experience, should be central to CPD and that formal educational provision, being only a small aspect of lifelong learning, should be complementary to and supportive of this[8,31,33]. Picking up the theme of experience-based learning, Cervero[34] points out that professionals' practice is characterised by 'complexities, uncertainties and conflicting values' (p. 85), which is one reason why traditional, didactic approaches to CPD are often inadequate – they fail to deal with the specific problems associated with any individual's practice. Nowlem[20] and Schon[35] both argue that, due to their in-depth knowledge of the practice setting, peers and colleagues should act as educators, and Schon proposes that they should adopt a coaching-type role: explaining what they would do in any given circumstance and the theoretical framework underlying their proposed choice of action. Much work has been conducted exploring different approaches to experience-based ('experiential') learning and examples of some of these, together with a discussion of their respective strengths and weaknesses and of assessment and validation issues, can be found in our paper: *Approaches to experiential learning in medicine. A background document*[36].

A great deal of discussion has also centred around those concepts of learning which are currently in vogue, such as Schon's notion of 'reflection-in-action' (discussed at length by Rogers[33] and also around various definitions of elements and stages of learning, such as Houle[37], which discusses stages of inquiry, instruction and performance. While the majority of these discussions have raised useful theoretical points, it should be noted that most are rhetorical in nature. While the concepts and models they propose undeniably promote further discussions of the nature of CPD and the requirements of educational programmes, most have not yet been adequately tested for their usefulness. Irrespective of the strength of their philosophical and theoretical foundations, their value and thus also their promotion, is not evidence-based.

With respect to the relative importance and popularity of self-directed learning and formal educational activities, a range of each has been cited as constituting CPD. The following list is drawn from Gear *et al.*[8], Parboosingh & Thivierge[25], Stanley *et al.*[31], Shirriffs[38] and Stross[22].

Formal activities
- conferences;
- courses and educational meetings journal clubs;
- workshops and small group work.

Self-directed (informal) activities and materials
- journals and texts;
- audio/videotapes;
- computer-assisted learning;
- self-assessment programmes;
- teaching;
- research;
- practice audits;
- clinical traineeships;
- discussions with colleagues;
- authorship.

Evidence about individual learning preferences must be taken into account as important, since it has implications for whether or not people are encouraged to learn in groups or multiprofessionally, and whether they are encouraged to learn in certain ways.

Considerable variation has been found among doctors regarding which of these learning activities they prefer. For example, Gear et al.[8] found that 10% of their sample preferred formal learning activities and 31% informal ones, but that more than half (55%) preferred to be able to use a mixture of the two. However, results in this area have not been consistent. Durno & Gill[39], for example, find that only 18% of a sample of GPs thought lunchtime meetings to be an acceptable source of regular education (with most, interestingly, considering discussions with *hospital* doctors their most important source of information and education). Grant et al.[9] also found a high rate of GP attendance at meetings where *hospital* doctors were the teachers. Both Shirriffs[38] and Reedy[40] found traditional, formal activities to be the most popular amongst the doctors they sampled. This is also true of newly qualified GPs[9].

One possible approach to individual and practice development which has its roots in the professional culture of peer review and the educational culture of adult learning principles is the Fellowship by Assessment Programme of the Royal College of General Practitioners[41]. Fellowship by Assessment was adopted by the RCGP in July 1989. It allows practitioners who are members of the College of 5 years standing to submit themselves, at a time of their own choosing, for a rigorous performance-based audit in which all the standards are published in advance with the research basis for them. It has immediate attractions for those who subscribe to the principles of adult learning, since the standards are objective and the learner can prepare for as long as they like, take whatever advice they like from whomever they like, and take it at times of their own choosing.

The standards are all based on the care of patients in general practice, and there is no need for the GP to do anything at all outside his/her practice. Thus Fellowship can be achieved simply by really good patient care in the work setting. The system is also based on peer-review and every candidate is visited by three assessors, all of whom are normally Fellows of the College themselves. The lead assessor is chosen by the central Fellowship by Assessment Committee and the other members of the visiting team are Fellows, at least one of whom must be local and known to the applicant.

A particularly attractive feature is that, since the standard is objective, there is no question of norm referencing the pass mark, so as many general practitioners as can reach this standard will get the Fellowship. Numbers have risen steadily but, since such Fellows work in partnerships, the College estimates that about half a million patients are currently looked after in a general practice in which at least one partner has Fellowship by Assessment. Since some of the standards cross all parts of the practice this is likely to be improving patient care considerably. Furthermore, since all the standards are actually measurable, it follows that the College can be certain that, in those practices at least, those standards have actually been demonstrated.

The Fellowship by Assessment Programme also taps into the view that CME/CPD should be increasingly work-based, rather than being provided centrally. Such an approach can increase the relevance of CPD activity and ensure that it is constructive and appropriate for a given practice.

It would appear therefore that a variety of learning activities and methods can be considered as valid constituents of CPD and that providers of formal programmes have a range of possible options from which to choose. Which of these have been shown to be most effective will be discussed in Section 4 of this review.

One important point remains to be made. This concerns the call, heard with increasing frequency, for multiprofessional approaches to be taken to the provision of CPD. As yet there is minimal evidence for the effectiveness of such approaches – in this report only two studies involved more than a single profession, and in each case the professionals concerned all worked in the health care arena. Much more research is required into the experience and effectiveness of multiprofessional interventions before any justification for such a call can be made. It is incontrovertible that different professions must work effectively together. It has not yet been equally demonstrated that learning together is an effective tactic, over and above organisational improvements.

The recent survey of the educational needs of newly qualified GPs[9] shows that, while multiprofessional education is rejected by the vast majority, the same people endorse being taught by members of other professions in meetings aimed at GPs. So, while GPs do not want to learn with other professions, they are happy to learn from them.
Along similar lines, Bell's[42] report concludes that:

The evidence from the literature seems to indicate that the rhetoric of the proponents of shared learning is more powerful and persuasive than the reality of practice.

However, Bell also points out that multiprofessional learning is taking place, and this is occurring locally, in response to local needs and practice. This finding, that joint learning best occurs in relation to joint need identified in the course of practice, is reinforced by the confidential report on improving quality in general practice[43], of which the Appendix is one part.

2.4 Influences on CPD provision

Government policy has already been mentioned as one influence on the extent of provision of formal CPD programmes, but other factors also have a bearing on this, as well as on the educational quality of programmes. Two major influences, linked to government policy, are those relating to accreditation issues and to financial input.

As the Department of Health[3] points out, the CME schemes endorsed by the Royal Colleges are all based on systems of credit accumulation, with the achievement of minimum targets over a 5-year period leading to a certificate of re-accreditation (although given the evidence reviewed in this paper, the application of sanctions to those who fail to meet the target would be of minimal effect in facilitating a more productive approach towards an individual's CPD). This kind of approach is widespread in medicine across Europe[44] and is also found farther afield, such as in the MOCOMP (Maintenance of Competence) scheme in Canada[25]. While credit-bearing CPD schemes have increased the number and variety of programmes on offer to doctors, they have not always guaranteed their quality[45]. This is despite the setting of criteria which must be met if programmes are to be judged as suitable for recognition in terms of accreditation and funding. An example of such criteria are those required for approval under the Postgraduate Education Allowance Scheme in general practice. According to the British Postgraduate Medical Federation[46,47], in order to be accepted for accreditation and funding under this scheme, programmes must:

- present clear aims to potential participants;
- demonstrate their relevance to the educational needs of practising GPs;
- be structured and include varied learning approaches;
- be able to cater for the varying needs of participants and provide individual feedback;
- give details of their evaluation.

Such programmes must also provide evidence that they are not promoting any treatment or approach in which the provider or sponsor has a financial interest.

A further factor of importance concerns the context of CME/CPD for credit-bearing programmes. In particular, the current evidence-based medicine movement has resulted in many such courses. Debates about the validity and value of this approach are not relevant to this review. However, the relevance of 'evidence' to practice can only be established in the practice context and it will be shown in later sections that objectivity of evidence is nowhere cited as a factor which either facilitates participation in CPD or change in practice, even though a desire to keep up-to-date is important. Taking evidence into ordinary practice as that practice needs seems to be a main message. The content of CPD should be driven by need rather than externally referenced factors.

In addition to the issue of quality, questions have also been raised regarding the value of credit accumulation schemes and their actual purpose. Grant[47] asks why the credit-bearing CME system is in place and what it is designed to achieve:

- to deal with bad apples?
- to prove CME is taking place?
- to develop new approaches to CME?
- as a response to a culture of managerialism?
- accountability and control?
- to ensure that learning opportunities are there?
- to support doctors?

The development by the General Medical Council of procedures to deal with poorly performing doctors has largely nullified the need to deal with the 'bad apple' question by means of CPD. Likewise, 'remedial training' cannot easily be seen as a role for CME/CPD systems.

In a survey of 125 professional bodies, Vaughan[1] found that much actual CPD is not credit-bearing and is likely to remain so. This view is supported by Gear et al.[8] who point out that much of CPD is difficult for professional bodies to recognise and reward, as it is self-directed and informal in nature. They propose that, while attempts should be made to increase the recognition of such learning, some will inevitably 'slip through the net' and they propose that learning of this nature should simply be considered a normal part of professional working life. The challenge that faces the profession is to recognise that this is a powerful form of life-long learning. Most of this cannot be measured in the form of events: learning in the context of practice is a continuous event best acknowledged through processes rather than events. Likewise, time for reflection on practice and on learning is important and cannot be measured in the same way as attendance at a lecture[48]. All of this does raise the question of what exactly CPD is as well as what credits actually represent, and there is a danger, as Cervero[34] suggests, that participation in educational programmes may become the primary goal of credit-bearing schemes, rather than learning itself.

In the light of the difficulties associated with such schemes, Grant[47] argues that systems based on the accumulation of credits or points may not be the most appropriate. She suggests that locally managed systems based on the developmental needs of particular units and of the doctors working in them (not excluding non-specific or general professional CME) may be more meaningful in terms of ensuring optimal patient care outcomes. In parallel, the Department of Health[3] proposes that health outcomes should be the criteria against which any investment in CME (in terms of both money and time) should be measured. They acknowledge that there is, as yet, no satisfactory method of doing this, but propose certain, interlinked roles and responsibilities of individuals, service managers and the Royal Colleges:

- individuals are responsible for devoting their time to maintaining their own competence;
- managers are responsible for ensuring that the necessary resources are available to enable individuals to do this;
- the Royal Colleges are responsible for setting standards and, in some instances, for contributing towards costs;
- Trusts also have a responsibility with respect to demonstrating their commitment to staff and promoting multidisciplinary programmes (whether or not this is wise)[49].

Another way of dealing with the question of value for money has been put forward by Hollwitz & Danielson[50], who suggest that financial values and benefits should be assigned to specific interventions, aimed at particular jobs and job functions, in order to foster cost-effective quality assurance. Having said this, however, it must be acknowledged that such types of cost-benefit are only one aspect of the overall professional agenda for learning, albeit an important one.

2.5 Influences on participation in CPD programmes

A number of studies have focused on the extent to which doctors and others participate in CPD programmes, with particular emphasis being placed on those factors which motivate or facilitate their participation and on those which deter them or act as barriers. Some motivating and facilitating factors which have been isolated are given in Table 1, where it can be seen that a general desire to keep up-to-date is the most commonly cited motivator

AUTHORS (and dates)	MOTIVATING/FACILITATING FACTORS ISOLATED
Cividin & Ottoson[73]	perceived need to confirm or alter current practices the chance to network with others
Byres et al.[105] Gear et al.[8]	satisfaction with previous courses/programmes attended the presence of a climate conducive to learning (arising from the Professional Body and prevailing throughout the profession)
Department of Health[3]	a need to keep up-to-date career changes (e.g. of specialty)
Vaughan[1]	to become/stay up-to-date to train for new, additional roles to increase job satisfaction and personal effectiveness
Woolf[106]	interest it the topics covered (found to be a much stronger motivator than perceived weaknesses)
Fox et al.[75]	a desire for competence (24%) pressure to change arising from the clinical environment (14%) financial incentives (9%)
Wood & Byrne[107]	a desire among GP's to escape from problems associated with their practices a desire to communicate with other GP's and other health professionals a hope for intellectual stimulation a general desire to keep up-to-date a need to refresh the memory and increase confidence
Barham & Benseman[108] and Gross[109]	working in group settings
Grant et al.[9]	need identified from practice, e.g. management training peer contact keeping up-to-date general interest

Table 1 Factors which motivate or facilitate participation in CPD.

for participation in CPD programmes, and that the opportunity for discussions with colleagues is another common positive influence. These non-instrumental, but highly professional factors must not be lost in future planning. Factors relating to professional competence are also frequently cited. Other influences of note are financial incentives, and satisfaction with programmes attended in the past. The effects of financial incentives were further investigated by Kelly & Murray[52] who studied GPs' reasons for attending postgraduate meetings, in relation to the introduction of the PGEA (Postgraduate Education Allowance which links a certain amount of GP's salary to proof of undertaking CME). They found that, while general interest remained a prime motivating factor (cited in 43% of cases), over a third of attenders (35%) gave the PGEA as a reason for their participation, while only 29% said that they were motivated by a desire to improve their knowledge, with only 0.4% giving a need to change their practice as a reason for attending. This proportion was half that made up by those who said that they did not know why they were there (0.8%)! More encouragingly, the 1998 survey by Grant *et al.* shows that young doctors do reflect on their practice and identify learning needs accordingly.

Making participation in programmes mandatory does not seem to have a great deal of effect on participation rates – Cervero[34,53] contends that there are small but insignificant increases only – and the practice has been found to have detrimental effects on participants' satisfaction with the programmes and also on their intentions with respect to future attendance at voluntary courses[54]. Furthermore, Walton[55] found that changes to practice are considered more satisfying if they are perceived to have arisen from reasons of personal incentive rather than from external pressures. Jones & Fear[56] found 'overwhelming opposition' to compulsory attendance at CPD programmes by human resources professionals in Wales, although some certification and recognition of CPD activities was welcomed by them.

A variety of barriers and deterrents to participation in CPD programmes have also been isolated. For example, differences between trainers and trainees, in terms of their learning styles, have been presented as a possible deterrent, although the evidence for this is tentative[57]. Other factors, however, are based on more conclusive evidence:

- the costs involved in terms of money and time[13,58];
- dissatisfaction with the quality of programmes on offer and a lack of personal benefit from participation[34,58];
- general apathy with respect to education[34];
- a preference for self-directed learning[34].

Finally, Branthwaite *et al.*[27] found regular attenders (GPs) at CPD meetings to be more progressive in their work than those who did not attending regularly, to be more concerned about developing their skills and about having the time and scope to practice effectively, and to be more conscientious with respect to developing and improving their work. Commenting on this paper, Gray[29] raises the question of whether the educational intervention had somehow promoted the development of these characteristics or whether people with such characteristics are those who are more motivated to seek out education.

Gray's question is just one of many which have been raised in connection with the outcomes of CPD, and an in-depth discussion of the findings of outcome studies and of effective educational strategies will follow. There are, however, numerous and complex methodological issues involved in the investigation of the effectiveness of CPD, and as these need to be taken into account if critical appraisal of outcome studies is to be fully informed, they will be dealt with first.

METHODOLOGICAL ISSUES

Studies investigating the effectiveness of CPD have frequently failed to do so in a conclusive manner[16,59,60] and a commonly cited reason for this lack of conclusiveness is that many such studies rest on weak methodological foundations[16,61,62]. Methodological difficulties have been found in a variety of areas, but are most notable in connection with design issues, with the influence of intervening variables, and with the measurement of outcomes.

3.1 The problem of design

3.1.1 Educational programme design

Problems associated with design fall into two categories: the design of educational programmes and the design of outcome studies. Firstly, with respect to formal CPD programmes, many of these have been shown to fail to identify the needs of learners and/or their client groups: a problem which often results in the further failure of programme designers to identify and define clear, relevant and measurable objectives[21,63,64]. One example of the latter problem is provided by a study (which, for obvious reasons, will not be cited) which gave its aim as being to investigate the effectiveness of management training for hospital doctors. The objectives of the study were presented as: the personal growth and development of participants and an improvement in the extent of their insight into their personal attitudes – very clear, very relevant and very measurable!

3.1.2 The design of outcome studies

With respect to the design of outcome studies themselves, Allery et al.[16] have raised the following criticisms:

- they frequently fail to use control groups or randomisation;
- statistical analysis of data is often inadequate;
- issues of validity are frequently ignored;
- many studies are correlational and/or retrospective (and are thus unhelpful in terms of increasing the understanding of causal processes).

However, Jacobson et al.[65] in their area argue powerfully that:

The randomised controlled trial alone reflects a reductionist approach that fails to do justice to the philosophy of general practice. The art of medicine is founded as context, anecdote, patient stories of illness and personal experience, and we should continue to blend this with good quality and appropriate research findings in patient care.

We shall see that such considerations are not irrelevant to educational research in medicine.

Other related criticisms of outcome studies tend to be related to the difficulties inherent in attempting to isolate the influences of particular activities from those of intervening variables and to problems connected with the measurement of outcomes. Both of these issues will shortly be discussed in depth but before this, consideration will be given to one type of outcome study which has generally been received with a considerable degree of acclaim: the randomised controlled study which, making reference to the large numbers of participants which are usually involved, Charlton[66] terms 'megatrials'. Because of their use of control groups and randomisation techniques, such studies are generally considered to fulfil the requirements of 'good science'[66] and they are therefore also widely considered to produce findings of guaranteed reliability. However, even this type of study is not immune to criticism. For example, Davis et al.[62], who conducted a review of 50 randomised controlled trials, have criticised them on the following grounds:

- they give too few details about participants;
- they give too few qualitative details;

- they too often use volunteer participants;
- they too rarely use 'blind' assessment (where assessors are ignorant of the experimental conditions to which individual participants have been assigned).

Charlton has also criticised this type of study, but on the grounds that they involve the deliberate recruitment of large, heterogeneous groups of participants and the averaging of findings across these large groups – a practice which he claims is not only of no value, but can also be dangerously misleading (p. 430):

On formal methodological grounds, an estimate of therapeutic effect derived from a megatrial tells the clinician nothing about the experiences of the individual subjects in that trial: a moderate average improvement may summarise many combinations of benefits, harms and no effect among trial participants.

Charlton raised these problems with specific reference to drug trials, but his points can nevertheless be applied to the assessment of the effects of educational activities: a moderate *average* improvement in performance across a large sample of practitioners could (assuming that none suffered a decline in performance as a result of the activity!) have been produced by a combination of a small number of large improvements and a larger number of 'no change' results. Were this to be the case, the findings would say nothing about the reasons for the effectiveness or non-effectiveness of the activity with respect to any individual practitioner's knowledge or performance. A further point which has been raised by Davis *et al.* and by Charlton is that randomised controlled trials cannot serve as tests of previously generated hypotheses, but are merely hypothesis-generating exercises themselves, with Charlton describing them as being an example of 'epistemological techniques'.

Despite having conducted their review, Davis *et al.* question the validity of making such cross-comparisons because of the inherent variations between trials. Beaudry[12,67,69] also questions the practice, but for reasons connected with the wide use of unstandardized assessment measures and, in relation to CME programmes, because of the 20% average dropout rate.

A final point which has been raised in connection with large-scale studies is mentioned by Moore[30], who points out that it is generally such large-scale and well-funded studies which manage to demonstrate the success of educational programmes. He argues that studies designed and conducted by the average CME office cannot match the scope of these large-scale studies and that they are therefore unlikely, however, well designed, to be able to replicate their findings.

3.2 The problem of intervening variables

Wergin *et al.*[70] suggest that as educational activities are not isolated events they should ideally be considered in relation to contextual influences. This view is reinforced by those studies which have shown that practitioners' behaviour can change as a result of factors which are, or appear to be, unrelated to educational intervention. Walton[55], for example, found that learning was perceived to be instrumental in doctors' behaviour change in only two-thirds of cases, while Allery *et al.*[16] found only half of this proportion (i.e. one-third) to be perceived as having been influenced by educational activity. Taking contextual influences into account is not an easy task, but, as Todd[10] has pointed out, it is extremely difficult to isolate particular interventions or actions as leading to goal achievement, and one of the reasons for this difficulty is the multiplicity of variables which may intervene at various stages of the process. With the expansion of CME into CPD, these problems have multiplied, as many of the informal, self-directed activities now carried out by learners are even more difficult to isolate in terms of their effects[8]. Figure 1 is an illustration of some of the variables which might intervene in the CPD process and the points in the process at which they might do this. Whilst only including a few examples of the huge range of variables which have the potential to intervene at the different stages of the CPD process, this diagram clearly

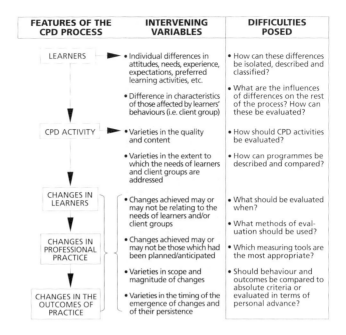

FEATURES OF THE CPD PROCESS	INTERVENING VARIABLES	DIFFICULTIES POSED
LEARNERS	• Individual differences in attitudes, needs, experience, expectations, preferred learning activities, etc.	• How can these differences be isolated, described and classified?
	• Difference in characteristics of those affected by learners' behaviours (i.e. client group)	• What are the influences of differences on the rest of the process? How can these be evaluated?
CPD ACTIVITY	• Varieties in the quality and content	• How should CPD activities be evaluated?
	• Varieties in the extent to which the needs of learners and client groups are addressed	• How can programmes be described and compared?
CHANGES IN LEARNERS	• Changes achieved may or may not be relating to the needs of learners and/or client groups	• What should be evaluated when?
		• What methods of evaluation should be used?
CHANGES IN PROFESSIONAL PRACTICE	• Changes achieved may or may not be those which had been planned/anticipated	• Which measuring tools are the most appropriate?
	• Varieties in scope and magnitude of changes	• Should behaviour and outcomes be compared to absolute criteria or evaluated in terms of personal advance?
CHANGES IN THE OUTCOMES OF PRACTICE	• Varieties in the timing of the emergence of changes and of their persistence	

Figure 1 Diagram to illustrate the difficulties posed by variables which may intervene in the CPD process.

illustrates the complexity, if not the impossibility, of trying to evaluate the influence of an educational activity with respect to professional behaviour or practice outcomes – whether or not the influence of contextual variables is acknowledged by those attempting the evaluation. While it might be possible to establish the causal processes in operation in very general terms, these cannot be predicted for any individual participant, and this circumstance severely impedes the efforts of those attempting to discover the means by which particular changes in practice, or in the outcomes of practice, might best be effected.

3.3 The problem of measurement

The difficulties facing researchers attempting to evaluate the effectiveness of CPD are further compounded by problems associated with the measurement of the outcomes of particular CPD activities. Van der Vleuten[71] suggests that the area of educational achievement testing is one which is 'in turmoil'. The extent of the problem was highlighted 20 years ago by Bertram & Brooks-Bertram[64]: having conducted their review of 66 studies of CME outcomes, they considered inadequate assessment to be one of the chief reasons for the failure of studies to demonstrate effectiveness in relation to CME programmes. The problems associated with the measurement of outcomes are 3-fold in nature, and concern:

- the type of outcome(s) to be measured;
- the most appropriate method(s) and tool(s) to use;
- the timing of the measurement in relation to the timing of the learning.

3.3.1 What should be measured?

One of the main problems with many of the studies which ostensibly concern themselves with the outcomes of CPD is that the outcomes they choose to study are not connected, or are only very loosely connected, with the aims of CPD, i.e. they fail to address the issues of changes in practice and in practice outcomes. The literature search conducted for the purpose of this review elicited many studies which involved the measurement of a wide range of such 'outcomes', and these are listed below:

- staff recruitment outcomes;
- scores on 'happiness indexes';
- changes in doctors' confidence;
- changes in levels of peer support;
- changes in the cost of staff training;
- further dissemination of knowledge;
- the intellectual stimulation of programmes;
- changes in participants' attitudes, values and beliefs;
- when and how CME was used during a period of change;
- whether participants' expectations of a programme were met;
- the extent to which participants had felt challenged by an educational programme;
- participants' satisfaction with the type, content and quality of programmes on offer;
- whether participants considered the benefits gained from a programme to have been worth the time invested in attending;
- the types and number of educational meetings attended, and the amount of time expended in attending these.

It would appear that some of the designers of these studies may have fallen into the trap outlined by Dall'Alba & Sandberg[69], p. 432):

In complex fields of practice, there is a risk that assessment highlights the readily measurable, over-emphasising detail, rather than promoting essential aspects of competence. In this way, practice is trivialised through assessment which fails to support competence development.

Others, however, *have assessed* factors directly related to the aims of CPD. Many studies, for example, have included an increase in practitioner knowledge as an outcome measure (and this might reasonably be presumed to be a prerequisite to changes in practice, even if these do not necessarily follow from it) and the majority have included measures of changes in types of behaviour or level of performance. Some examples of these are listed below:

- general clinical management;
- use of investigations;
- prescribing practices;
- counselling strategies;
- use of screening techniques and preventive care practices;
- diagnostic accuracy;
- referral practices;
- follow-up consultations.

It should be noted that practitioners' perceptions of changes in their own performance do not always provide accurate reflections of actual change and that studies investigating changes in practice do not always distinguish between the two[72].

The assessment of patient outcomes is less common than the assessment of doctors' professional performance but, despite this, considerable breadth in the type of indicators selected can be seen in the list of examples from the literature given below:

- safety (in relation to anaesthesia);
- perceptions of care received;
- increased coping skills;
- emotional well-being;
- understanding of conditions experienced;
- mortality rates;
- increased self-efficacy;
- Caesarean birth rates.

One point which ought to be raised here is whether, in the light of the factors which researchers consider important to investigate in relation to formal CPD provision, the aims of CPD are sufficiently inclusive. One argument supporting the possibility that they are not is that a frequent (and perfectly acceptable) outcome of CME is that doctors take an informed decision not to make any change to their practice[25,73]. The general assumption that change in practice is always required and improvement in competence always possible may be ignoring the facts: given the amount of time and effort spent in undergraduate and postgraduate training by all doctors, there are bound to be areas of their practice in which their practices are already up-to-date and in which they are fully competent. (Davis *et al.*[74] propose a ceiling effect to be generally operating with respect to the management of hypertension.) It would be worrying were this not the case. It must therefore be true, as Fox *et al.*[75] point out, that changes in behaviour are not always necessary, and that some changes which do occur are too small to be measured.

Finally, consideration must be given to why some CPD activities do appear to be ineffective. Little published attention has been paid to this, although Davis *et al.*[74] did put forward some possible explanations for the apparent ineffectiveness of some activities: that the changes produced are too small to be noted by the methods of assessment used; that ceiling effects are operating (such as in the management of hypertension); and that variations across practitioners, settings and behaviours (caused by multiple intervening variables) lead to the appearance of no effect when results are averaged, as in randomised controlled trials. The methodological problems outlined in Section 3.1 and 3.2 of this report will also hamper these efforts.

3.3.2 What methods and tools should be used?
A wide variety of methods and tools of assessment and evaluation have been used in studies of the effectiveness of CPD. In terms of the assessment of patient outcomes, these usually involve one or more of the following: clinical audit techniques, health assessment scales or questionnaires, and occasionally, knowledge quizzes. With respect to professionals' performance, there appear to be at least as many methods and tools of assessment available for assessors to choose from as there are theories of learning. A small selection are given below:

- checklists;
- self-assessment tests;
- peer review self-report questionnaires;
- chart audits;
- competence-based methods rating scales;
- computer diaries;
- criterion-referenced methods;
- credit accumulation;
- multiple choice tests;
- learning portfolios.

Each method and type of tool has its own advantages and disadvantages in terms of their reliability and validity, their generalizability and their feasibility (in terms of the time required for evaluation, etc.). Despite these differences, very few studies attempt to compare or even discuss different methods or tools in terms of these characteristics. (However, the 'Good Assessment Guide'[76] provides a useful comparative description of them in relation to each individual method as used within medical education.) Reasons for this are related, firstly, to the difficulty in establishing reliability and validity (which usually involves large numbers of participants and complicated standardisation procedures), and, secondly, to the need to test each participant by means of a variety of time-consuming methods in order for reliability not to be compromised as a result of content specificity problems (the variation displayed by individual learners across different tasks[70].

The advantages and disadvantages of adopting any particular method or tool need to be weighed up within the situational and institutional contexts of the evaluation, with selection depending on the educational environment, the resources available, the attitudes of learners and teacher or trainers, and so on[77]. In practice, although there are a number of standardised measures available[3], many evaluations involve the use of unstandardized ones[12], and these may be specifically designed for particular studies[45]. However, as Van der Vleuten argues, no single method or tool is a panacea in the assessment of performance, and the content and relevance of tasks to the context of practice and the outcomes to be tapped are more important than the validity of the particular instruments selected for use. What is crucial, he argues, is that those who are being assessed are presented with educationally and professionally valid challenges.

Benett's[78] point should also be taken into account here: that work-based professional standards are not absolute, but are established, maintained and improved by means of negotiation and professional pragmatism. Therefore, all methods and measures ought to be regularly reviewed[70] and the expenditure of a great deal of time and effort on the development of measures may not be appropriate. In connection with this issue, Van der Vleuten has also contested the current popularity of objective measures and the fact that many now consider them to be, by definition, superior to more subjective measurement techniques[79]. This stance is contested on two grounds: firstly, on the basis that objective measurement methods do not necessarily produce more reliable results than subjective ones, and, secondly, on the basis that reproducibility of findings is a more useful goal of measurement than objectivity per se, and that the influence of subjective error on reproducibility is limited. The use of subjective measures also removes the need for large-scale validation and standardisation studies.

The Good CME Guide (1998) offers a variety of methods of demonstrating the benefit of CME activity to individual doctors and to the institution. The methods are feasible and derive from the ways in which doctors actually improve and judge their own practice and its effects.

3.3.3 When should effectiveness of CPD be evaluated?
The timing of the evaluation of the outcomes of CPD activities in relation to the timing of those activities is something which has not received a great deal of attention in the literature, but is an issue in need of some consideration. As Gibbs et al.[80] found, perceptions of the value of educational experience change over time: the 'feel good' factor has a tendency to decrease on participants' return to work where the benefits of newly acquired knowledge and skills may not be immediately apparent. Boud[81] suggests that an initial evaluation may need to include the identity and exploration of feelings engendered by the experience of the CPD activity so that these cannot then bias later evaluations. Al-Shehri et al.[72] propose that indications of the feature(s) of an activity participants later find useful in practice can be addressed within a 'reasonable period' after the activity has taken place – unfortunately they do not specify what constitutes a reasonable period. The sparseness of information in this area suggests a need for further research into the timing and persistence of the outcomes of CPD activities in relation to the timing of the activities themselves.

Taking all these methodological issues together, it can clearly be seen that the evaluation of the effectiveness of CPD is a far from simple task and that there are many difficulties and complexities facing the researcher in this field. This background of confused definitions, confused aims and outcomes, and widely varying methods and tools of assessment must be kept in mind during any consideration of the findings of the outcome studies in this field.

FINDINGS OF THE REVIEW

For the purpose of this review, the following databases were searched for journal articles published from 1990 onwards:

- BIDS (Bath Information and Data Service);
- Social Science Citation Index;
- Medline;
- First Search;
- ERIC (Educational Resources and Information Centre);
- Current Index of Journals in Education.

Keywords used included: continuing medical education; continuing professional development; nurse education; health professional education; evaluation; outcome measures.

In total, 2561 articles were found in connection with CME and CPD, but of these only 118 remained when 'outcome' was added as a search item. Sixty-two of these 118 papers reported studies in connection with the medical profession, 36 related to nursing and allied professions (e.g. health visiting) and 20 to other professions. The criteria for studies to be included in this report were that the outcomes they assessed were connected with patient care, practitioner knowledge or practitioner behaviour/performance. As reported earlier, few studies which purport to investigate the outcomes of CPD address themselves directly to the attainment of its aims and this was reflected by the result of applying these criteria to the 118 outcome studies elicited by the search: only 16 remained for consideration. Of these 16 studies, six involved doctors, six involved nurses or members of allied professions, one involved both doctors and nurses and one was multidisciplinary. Only one study did not concern health care practitioners and that involved college staff. Thirteen studies considered practitioner outcomes alone, one considered patient outcomes alone, and two considered both. It must be remembered that the references cited do include two review articles by Davis et al.[64,75].

Reflecting the broadening of views concerning the types of activities which constitute CPD, a wide range of such activities can be observed in the studies reviewed, including not only formal programmes and conferences, but also teleconferencing, collaborative study groups, audio/videotapes and slides, behavioural approaches, problem-based methods, practice guidelines and newsletters. Measurement of outcomes involved the use of questionnaires, document reviews (e.g. involving patients' medical notes), written tests of knowledge and attitudes, self-reports, the judgements of experts (e.g. with respect to diagnostic accuracy), direct observation and interviews.

4.1 The extent to which CPD aims were achieved

The literature only offers evidence (as opposed to discussion) about formal CME/CPD events rather than about on-going practice-based, individual CPD based on reflection and experience. The following review of evidence must be interpreted in this light, and should not be seen as promoting that view of CPD. The effects of creating and managing learning opportunities within everyday professional life have not been addressed in the research literature: for example, learning from patients, case discussions, referral letters, effects of the management of patients, in-practice reviews and discussion with colleagues. It is important to recognise these ways of continuing to learn and refine them, making them more conscious and purposeful as the basis of a professionals approach to lifelong learning. However, the literature is inadequate in addressing these methods.

4.1.1 Results in connection with patient outcomes

All three of the studies which reported practitioners' use of activities aimed at patient outcomes found improvements to have occurred as a result of those activities. In the first of these studies, patients with breast cancer who were cared for by nurses who had undergone a training programme on the subject reported more positive perceptions of the care they received than did a control group and they also displayed a greater level of knowledge about their condition and lower anxiety levels[82]. The differences were found to be statistically significant in each case. Gerrard et al.[83] found that training health visitors in the detection, treatment and prevention of postnatal depression had a positive influence on the emotional well-being of their clients.

The third study showing improvements in patient outcomes[84] reported the effects of a collaborative study group which aimed to improve patient care by monitoring the outcomes of coronary artery by-pass graft (CABG) operations across institutions in northern New England. The group met at least three times a year and operated in the following ways:

- information was disseminated by newsletter to all members of the group between meetings;
- all members were trained in the use of quality improvement tools and techniques;
- members conducted a comparative process analysis in order to learn about best practices.

The study found that average in-hospital mortality in relation to CABG had decreased significantly in the 3 years since the group had been established. The group had also discovered the most common cause of death following CABG across the hospitals in the region and a further study was being conducted to try to discover why this problem was occurring and what improvements could be made to patient care in order to reduce its incidence and/or lessen the severity of its consequences.

4.1.2 Results in connection with practitioner outcomes

Thirteen of the 15 studies concerned with practitioner outcomes claimed to have achieved positive changes in knowledge, behaviour and/or performance, with the findings of the other two being inconclusive. Statistical analysis of findings was not possible or appropriate in all cases, but significance was claimed in four studies[82,85,86,87]. Change had been found in relation to a wide range of topics and behaviours, as can be seen from the list presented below:

- collaborative care and multidisciplinary working;
- prescription practices;
- knowledge and practices relating to pain management;
- knowledge of health promotion issues;
- practitioners' health-related behaviour;
- expansion of practitioners' professional roles;
- the 'timely application' of theory to practice diagnostic accuracy (two studies);
- referral practices;
- changes to teaching strategies and curriculum planning;
- the detection, treatment and prevention of postnatal depression;
- knowledge relating to gerontology;
- knowledge and practices relating to cardiac arrhythmias;
- knowledge and practices relating to breast cancer nursing.

Four studies were found to have achieved particularly interesting findings and these will therefore be discussed in more detail. Two of these[86,88] raised issues connected with variations in outcome across participants and the need for contextual factors to be considered in connection with outcomes.

Mann et al.'s paper reports the outcomes of a problem-based training programme concerned with the promotion of cardiac health. The programme involved practitioners based at three different worksites and coming from a variety of professions related to health care (including doctors, nurses, dieticians, pharmacists and social workers[89]. The goals of the study were: to promote collaborative care and multidisciplinary working, to increase up-to-date and specific knowledge, to increase awareness of available resources, and to increase practitioners' skills with respect to changing other people's behaviour. All goals were met in all sites, but there were clear variations in the extent to which change took place, or was perceived to have taken place, across the three sites (for example, in the extent to which interdisciplinary collaboration was fostered) and between disciplines (for example, in all areas except community development and health promotion, physicians were the least likely professional group to perceive that they had learned anything). These differences raise the question of the context in which training takes place. Given the interdisciplinary nature of this programme it is likely that most participants would be relatively uninformed at the outset in relation to some areas about which information was presented. In such circumstances, the level at which the information would need to be pitched would probably not be sufficiently high for physicians to gain very much except in those areas with which they would not themselves be very familiar, and these were likely to have been fewer in number than those with which the members of other professions were unfamiliar.

Crandall's study[88] was based on a qualitative case study approach and followed the practice of five doctors for a period of six months after they had attended a 1-day conference on cardiac arrhythmias. Although the conference organisers had aimed to promote changes in practice, this objective had not been made explicit to those attending the conference. Three of the five doctors studied committed themselves, on the day of the conference, to making changes to their practice, while a fourth later made a decision to do so. Of the nine changes the doctors had committed themselves to making, six were still being practiced six months later. However, the differences between the participants, in terms of both decisions to change practice and actual changes made, prompted Crandall to state that:

CME does make a difference, but programme planners must pay attention to the circumstances under which it does.(p. 346)

The findings of these two studies underline the influence of intervening variables and the problems associated with trying to isolate their effects from those of CPD activities.

Dalton's study[90] highlighted the importance of the timing of evaluations of the effectiveness of CPD activities and the need for gains in participants' knowledge to be followed up so that any consequent changes in practice might be observed. The study concerned the results of an educational programme which was designed to increase nurses' knowledge in connection with pain management and which anticipated that increases in knowledge would lead to changes in practice. The programme did not significantly increase the knowledge of the participating nurses but, despite this, changes in practice which were attributed to the programme, were seen to emerge about 6 months after its completion. These changes involved increased documentation (e.g. of pain intensity ratings and anxiety levels) and improved prescribing practices. This study shows that the evaluation of the effectiveness of CPD activities needs therefore to be carefully conducted in order to assess the magnitude and scope of their effects – as this study has shown, small initial changes may have consequences beyond those which might have been expected. Further research is required into the time-span over which the consequences of particular activities may become apparent, together with any contextual influences on this.

The fourth study of particular interest was that of De Buda & Woolf[91]. The intervention outlined in this paper ('Saturday at the University') was a series of single-day events for family physicians which covered three Saturdays in the spring and another three in the autumn of three consecutive years. The paper reports on the effectiveness of the programme as judged at the end of the first year. The reason this study is of interest is that it demonstrates that formal educational programmes aimed at large numbers of participants are not necessarily ineffective (despite the extent of the criticism which has been directed towards them). Each of the 'Saturday at the University' training days used the same format, involving a series of 10-minute presentations, each of which was followed by 10 minutes of questions (some written and some from 'the floor'). Each major topic covered involved a series of presentations by the same person and each presentation focused on just three main points, which were reinforced by handouts. Participants were also given paper copies of all slides used in presentations. Evaluation of the outcomes of this programme was by means of a self-report postal questionnaire sent out to doctors three months after they had attended the last of the six days which comprised the first year of the course. Ninety-three per cent of respondents said that they had gained in knowledge and that they were applying their new knowledge to the care and management of their patients. Possibly because the findings were based on self-reports, De Buda & Woolf[91] were quite tentative in claiming the effectiveness of the programme, concluding (p. 283):

There is evidence that a single CME activity might not result in change[75] but may help to prepare for change, and it is likely that this was achieved by Saturday at the University.

The authors did, however, put forward several suggestions for the apparent success of this programme and these will be discussed in the next part of this paper, together with other factors which have emerged, both from this report and from earlier studies, as enhancing the effectiveness of the CPD process.

4.2 Influences on the effectiveness of the CPD process

Several of those whose work has been reviewed here have proffered suggestions as to the reasons underlying the relative success of their programmes, and these are given in Table 2. The importance of the accurate assessment of need was raised in nearly all of the studies reviewed, and many propose it as being the crucial first step in the planning of effective CPD activities[63,71,73,91]. This topic therefore warrants further discussion. Another area which will be discussed in some depth is concerned with those strategies and features which have been shown to enhance effectiveness across a range of different types of intervention.

AUTHORS (and dates)	SUGGESTIONS MADE
Hadiyono et al.[85]	That examples of good practice are established as normative behaviour amongst groups of colleagues
Kushnir et al.[110]	That speakers at formal presentations be expert in the field they are discussing
Malenka & O'Connor[84]	That a person of authority be in charge of educational programmes That, where cross-institutional collaboration is required, one person at each institution be responsible for the management of the intervention
Alexander[82]	That evaluation of the effectiveness of activities is an essential part of programme development That the evaluation of patient outcomes, while challenging, is an integral part of programme evaluation
Du Buda & Woolf[91]	That the development of good interpersonal relationships between participants be promoted

[1]Largely, that published from 1990 to date. This includes Davis et al.'s 1992 and 1995 reviews, but not original references to most of the papers they cite which were published before 1990. Their conclusions are, none the less, accepted and used.

[2]Due to the recency of the introduction of CPD as a term to describe ongoing professional learning, much of the literature refers to CPD or CME, and these terms will be used where they appear in the original papers.

Table 2 Education providers' perceptions of the reasons for their success.

4.2.1 The importance of needs assessment

Laxdal[4] and Davis & Thomson[93] describe learning needs in terms of gaps between ideal and actual practitioner performance, but others expand on this and argue that the needs of practitioners' client groups also be taken into account when CPD activities are planned[82]. It also seems logical that any deficiencies in terms of knowledge and understanding will need to be identified and rectified if such gaps are to be filled. Davis & Thomson[93] propose that effective needs assessment can promote the targeting of activities to the areas of need and the removal of barriers to change in the practice setting.

Laxdal[4] suggests that, although needs assessment is vital, it is poorly understood and difficult to do well, and that it is therefore often inadequately carried out. This view is supported by the findings of Williams et al.[94] who discovered that the usual method of analysis performed in relation to a standard needs assessment survey instrument (in terms of frequency counts and average scores for expressed preferences) would have led, if acted upon, to a series of courses heavily biased towards only one or two topics which would have disappointed more than half of those who had completed the survey. They found that factor analysis provided a more realistic picture. However, factor analysis is a difficult statistical technique and interpretation can be quite challenging, even if it has been carried out using a computer, and many would be deterred from attempting it on these grounds. Others may not have the resources to purchase the software required for computer analysis, which tends to be expensive.

One suggestion that has been raised in the literature is that practitioners should conduct their own needs assessment, possibly with the help of computerised diary packages[25], but others have questioned the reliability of this method. Davis & Thomson[93], for example, ask whether doctors are really able to judge their own competencies, and Chambers[7] argues that, in its extreme form, self-identification of learning needs:

....puts the onus on practitioners to solve the deep-rooted and vexed questions surrounding the relationships between theory and practice, subject knowledge and competence in these fields – thus absolving educators themselves of the need to continue to address such issues. (p. 16)

A possible solution which has been proposed to this problem is the use of the Delphi technique[95]. As Chambers explains, this technique involves the setting of a consensus regarding the competencies needed by members of a profession by a group of around 20 expert practitioners of that profession. Although the technique produces only a very general assessment of needs, the criteria, once established, can be used in the form of a questionnaire to help learners identify their own individual needs. Chambers does point out, however, that learners do not rate themselves as well as their educators do and that caution is therefore required. Tracey et al.[96] have also demonstrated the inaccuracy of GPs' self-assessments of knowledge. So even this essential element is not without its challenges.

Despite the heavy emphasis placed by authors on the importance of accurate needs assessment, few viable suggestions have been found with respect to how such accuracy might be achieved. The point made by the Department of Health in 1994 clearly still applies: there is a need for practical, effective and acceptable methods by which the learning needs of individual doctors can be objectively determined.

Having recognised the importance of needs assessment, one further factor must be considered: the question of whose needs? Learning or development needs will be assessed in the context of the practice and of quality of service to patients and the community. There are many formal ways of involving patients in such a needs assessment[97]. There are also models of needs assessment in primary care which are rooted in the consultation and have a patient orientation. The Canadian MOCOMP programme[25] is such a model. There are others, often less well known and less well evaluated. These include experiential learning, service-based learning, personal learning plans, learning contracts, portfolio-based learning, PUNs and DENs, self assessment, appraisal, peer-assessment and tutoring and competence-based assessment. These, and others, are discussed in Stanton & Grant[36].

It should also be remembered that, given unreliability, limited scope and frequent lack of practical feasibility of formal methods, needs assessment can be relatively informal, based on professional judgement and organisational development, and still just as effective. Grant et al.[11] have shown this, as have Fish & Coles[48]. The Lewisham model of CME planning[98] demonstrates a feasible approach towards individual and institutional needs assessment.

4.2.2 Effective strategies and features of CPD activities

Davis & Thomson[93] present a list of strategies in terms of the extent of their effectiveness in producing positive changes in performance, as follows.

Highly effective strategies
- practice-linked strategies;
- multifaceted strategies (especially those including three or more elements);
- academic outreach, e.g. promotion of rational prescribing behaviour by specially trained academics.

Moderately effective strategies
- audit/feedback (especially if individualised and presented by a person of authority);
- opinion leaders.

Ineffective strategies
- educational materials (especially unsolicited, printed material sent via the mail);
- formal CME (especially didactic courses).

The last 'ineffective' strategy, however, should not include short educational meetings with both didatic and interactive components[9].

Moore[30] has claimed that the changes which have recently taken place in the health care environment have resulted in positive new approaches in CPD, such as an increased emphasis on learning and on learning activities with direct relevance to clinical practice, the integration of CPD into the health care system, and an increase in cooperative planning of activities. An increased focus on research-based evidence regarding those features and strategies with a positive influence on the CPD process, rather than on the ongoing (and apparently self-perpetuating) rhetoric which is evident in much of the literature, is one way in which these changes in approach can be fostered and promoted.

Davis & Thomson[93] are strongly supportive of self-directed learning in preference to more formal activities, and give the following as their reason (p. 162):

There is already evidence that physicians exposed to self-directed learning, often co-ordinated through small-group, problem-based strategies continue their practice of self-directed learning, keeping up to date, later in practice.

However, Tracey et al.'s[96] findings do call into question the whole basics of self-directed learning and not all formal activities are ineffective, as the study by de Buda & Woolf[91] has demonstrated. A consideration of those features of activities which serve to enhance the effectiveness of both formal and self-directed activities may be more productive than a rigid endorsement of one type of activity over another.

The 1992[62] and 1995[74] reviews by Davis & Thomson and Davis et al., respectively, and Davis & Thomson's 1996[93] paper all point to the following features as being those which can enhance effectiveness:

- predisposing features – those which predispose individuals to change (e.g. those which impart information);
- enabling features – those which enable the change by facilitating its application in the practice environment (such as the rehearsal of desirable behaviours);
- reinforcing features – those which reinforce the change (e.g. reminders and feedback).

The influence of these features is further supported by the strong resemblance they bear to those incorporated into the PRECEDE-PROCEED model of behaviour change[99,100] which has been shown to be effective in relation to health promotion. In their 1992 review, Davis *et al.* found that, while activities incorporating predisposing features alone were moderately successful in terms of achieving improvements in performance, they were almost always ineffective with respect to improving patient outcomes. Where either enhancing or reinforcing features, or both, were combined with predisposing features, however, the effectiveness of the activities concerned was greatly enhanced. Davis *et al.*[74,101] concluded therefore that the most important positive influence on the CPD process was the use of practice-based, enabling and reinforcing strategies in conjunction with predisposing strategies and adequate needs assessment. At this point, it becomes clear that effective CPD must be seen as a process rather than an educational event.

This perhaps daunting conclusion was endorsed by the 1995 review and has also been supported by Ottoson[102] who incorporated the three types of features into her 'Application Process Framework' – a theoretical model of the stages involved in designing and planning a CPD programme. Ottoson, however, also stressed the importance of the context in which the elements of the programme were received by participants. Grilli & Lomas[103] have pointed out that innovations are adopted faster if they:

- represent only small departures from current practices;
- are not unduly complex;
- can be tried out in practice;
- are compatible with current thinking.

Gale & Grant's[17] research into the management of change in medicine supports these findings. They show that acceptance that there is a problem, recognition of the solution and support for the change are crucial. In addition, presenting the change as incremental and having demonstration of it are powerful tools.

The successful programme designed by De Buda & Woolf [91], while displaying features common to traditional, and often unsuccessful CME interventions (such as large numbers of participants and didactic presentations), can also be seen to display examples of those features described by Davis *et al.*[62] as being characteristic of effective activities. Firstly, the designers conducted a needs assessment in relation to the programme while it was still at the planning stage. Secondly, by limiting presentations to 10 minutes each, and by varying the type and pace of input by introduction of 10 minutes of questions between each presentation and the next, participants' attention to the predisposing elements of the course was enhanced, as was the likelihood of their retaining the information presented. The likelihood of the retention of information was further enhanced by the restriction placed on presentations to emphasise no more than three key points, salient to practice. The amount of time which was devoted to dealing with participants' questions (up to 200 were dealt with per day) could be considered an enhancing feature, and the programme handouts and notes served as a reinforcing features as participants reported having used them when needed in consultations with patients.

This consideration of De Buda & Woolf's[91] programme in terms of those features proposed as enhancers of the effectiveness of the CPD process, has rendered its success easily interpretable, and the importance of the features concerned has again been underlined.

An inspection of the suggestions made by the other providers of activities in the studies reviewed here (see Table 2) further supports the role of strategies which incorporate enabling and reinforcing features, as most of those described as possible enhancers of effectiveness could be described as one or other of these.

It is important to note here, then, that a practice-based and learner-orientated system of CME does not imply that the entire process should occur in the practice, nor that it should not contain a didactic element.

SUMMARY OF IMPORTANT ISSUES

The literature review has given rise to some important points which might be used for policy planning. They are reiterated here.

- Awareness has increased of the prevalence of self-directed learning among professionals and of the role this has to play in their ongoing development: most 'continuous learning' is likely to be initiated, organised, controlled and evaluated by the individual, and formal inputs play only a supporting, if important, role.
- It is important to note that self-directed learning implies only that the learners are in a position to decide what needs they have (deriving from their own, or their organisation's needs) and to play a major part in deciding what benefit has been derived from the CPD undertaken. That CPD, however, can take any acceptable and relevant form ranging from relatively traditional and formal to highly innovative and informal methods. The teaching and learning method is not the key variable.
- Three models of CME are commonly seen: 'update models' aim simply to communicate or disseminate information. There is a danger with this type of model that the acquisition of information may not be translated into improvements in practice. 'Competence models' aim to ensure that at least minimum standards for knowledge, skills, and attitudes are attained. Programmes based on this type of model may be sufficient to provoke alterations of practice, but they do not necessarily address the issue of whether such alterations lead to optimised patient care outcomes. 'Performance models' (which are beginning to gain prominence) aim not only to help doctors overcome barriers to successful changes in practice, but also to help them resolve clinical concerns.
- The objective measurement of the outcome of CME is usually too fraught with confounding variables and practical problems to be undertaken. However, demonstration of the benefit of CME, building on professional judgement is feasible and meaningful. Evidence suggests that individual doctors vary considerably in their preference for different learning methods. These preferences must be taken into account rather than adopting a rigid view of how doctors 'ought' to like to learn. Evidence suggests that learning method is less important than many other factors.
- While credit-bearing CPD schemes have increased the number and variety of programmes on offer to doctors, they have not always guaranteed their quality, relevance or effect.
- In addition to the issue of quality, questions have also been raised regarding the value of credit accumulation schemes on the grounds that they do not directly address the issue of patient care outcomes. This raises the question of what exactly CPD is as well as what credits actually represent. There is a danger that participation in educational programmes may become the primary goal of credit-bearing schemes, rather than learning itself.
- In the light of the difficulties associated with credit-based schemes, systems based on the accumulation of credits or points may not be the most appropriate. Locally managed systems based on the development needs of particular units and of the doctors working in them may be more meaningful in terms of ensuring optimal patient care outcomes.
- Much actual CPD is not credit bearing and is likely to remain so. This is difficult for professional bodies to recognise and reward, as it is self-directed and informal in nature. Attempts should be made to increase the recognition of such learning.
- Questions of value for money cannot be avoided. Although there are no satisfactory ways of doing this, a broad framework of responsibility should be established which is likely to increase cost-effectiveness. This will involve allocating responsibility for ensuring that the necessary resources are available; for setting standards; for contributing towards costs and to demonstrating commitment to CPD.
- Value for money will be increased when CME planning integrates both personal needs and interests and the development plans of organisations.
- Changes to practice are considered more satisfying if they are perceived to have arisen from reasons of personal incentive rather than from external pressures.

- Many formal CPD programmes fail to identify the needs of learners and/or their client groups, although it could be argued that responsibility for needs assessment is the learner's who then chooses what provision to accept.
- The huge range of variables which have the potential to intervene at the different stages of the CPD process illustrates the complexity, if not the impossibility, of trying to assess the influence of an educational activity on professional behaviour or practice outcomes – whether or not the influence of contextual variables is acknowledged by those attempting the evaluation. While it might be possible to establish the causal processes in operation in very general terms, these cannot be predicted for any individual participant, and this circumstance severely impedes the efforts of those attempting to discover the means by which particular changes in practice, or in the outcomes of practice might best be effected.
- In complex fields of practice, there is a risk that assessment highlights the readily measurable, over-emphasising detail rather than promoting essential aspects of competence. In this way, practice is trivialized through assessment which fails to support professional development.
- The general assumption that change in practice is always required and improvement in competence always possible may be ignoring the facts: given the amount of time and effort spent in undergraduate and postgraduate training by all doctors, there are bound to be vast areas of their practice which they are already up-to-date and in which they are fully competent. CPD might simply demonstrate this fact.
Work-based professional standards are not absolute, but are established, maintained and improved by means of negotiation and professional pragmatism.
- The timing of assessment of the outcomes of CPD activities in relation to the timing of the activities themselves is something which has not received a great deal of attention in the literature, but which is an issue in need of some consideration.
- CME does make a difference, but programme planners must pay attention to the circumstances under which it does. These may include:
    (a) predisposing features – those which predispose individuals to change (e.g. those which impart information);
    (b) enabling features – those which enable the change by facilitating its application in the practice environment (such as the rehearsal of desirable behaviours);
    (c) reinforcing features – those which reinforce the change (e.g. reminders and feedback);
    (d) assessment of the needs of practitioners and their clients/patients;
    (e) a consideration of the influence of relevant contextual factors.
- There is a need for practical, effective and acceptable methods by which the learning needs of individual doctors can be determined. Although needs assessment is vital, it is poorly understood and difficult to do well, and it is often inadequately carried out. Given the unreliability, limited scope and frequent lack of practical feasibility of formal methods, needs assessment can be relatively informal based on professional judgement and organisational development, and still be just as effective.
Innovations are adopted faster if they represent only small departures from current practices, if they are not unduly complex, if they can be tried out in practice and if they are compatible with current thinking.
- Available evidence all suggests that CPD should be developed as a process of planning, doing, and reviewing effect. Focusing on the nature and management of that process will be the most effective strategy.
- An increased focus on research-based evidence regarding those features and strategies with a positive influence on the CPD process, rather than on the ongoing (and apparently self-perpetuating) rhetoric about learning theories and learning methods which is evident in much of the literature, is one way in which changes in approach can be fostered and promoted. As yet there is minimal evidence for the effectiveness of some widely advocated approaches.

MOVING ON FROM HERE: A FOCUS ON PROCESS

The review has shown that there is no educational panacea, no 'most effective' learning method, no 'best buy' outcome measures. It has also shown that there is a more productive way of looking at the question of outcomes than seeking specific events and observable consequences. That more productive way involves looking at how the conditions for effectiveness of CPD activity (of whatever type) can be created. And that is by establishing a process and culture rather than specifying particular events, educational experiences or types of education or certain outcomes. It might be best to base conclusions about the outcomes of CPD on professional judgement, explicitly made and defended.

Our conclusion must be that the effectiveness of CPD is a function of the process and the context in which it occurs and not of one or another specific event or educational intervention in a professional life. We must therefore focus on improving the quality of the process and making it more relevant to individual needs and interests, service needs, the needs of the team and the practice. The process of planning and undertaking CPD must be managed so that those needs and interests are met, and outcomes can be judged in practical and professionally appropriate ways. CPD will therefore be a positive contribution to development. Different processes are used to identify and deal with poor performance – that cannot be a function of CPD.

In terms of development work, it can be proposed that:

- a wide range of acceptable and feasible approaches to needs assessment and CPD planning for the individual and the unit be developed and existing ones described, and supporting documentation provided;
- a wide range of appropriate methods of education or development be described;
- practical and professionally relevant guidelines for the reasonable evaluation of outcomes be prepared, based on professionally appropriate methods and explicit professional judgement.

Practices and practitioners demonstrating CME/CPD management processes, by implementing at least one of the suggested approaches from each stage, could receive due recognition and reward.

REFERENCES

1 Vaughan P. Maintaining professional competence: a survey of the role of professional bodies in the development of credit-bearing CPD courses. Hull: University of Hull; 1991.

2 Royal College of Obstetricians and Gynaecologists. CME credit book. London: Royal College of Obstetricians and Gynaecologists; 1994.

3 Department of Health. Consultation paper for the chief medical officer's conference on continuing education for doctors and dentists. Working document. Department of Health; 1995.

4 Laxdal OE. Needs assessment in continuing medical education: a practical guide. J Med Educ 1982;57:827-34.

5 Royal Australian College of General Practitioners. Quality Assurance and Continuing Education Programme 1993–95. Rozelle, NSW: Royal Australian College of General Practitioners; 1993.

6 Singleton A, Tylee A. Continuing medical education in mental illness: a paradox for general practitioners. Br J Gen Pract 1996;46:339-41.

7 Chambers E. Mentoring, self-directed learning, and continuing professional education. Milton Keynes: The Open University; 1992.

8 Gear J, McIntosh A, Squires G. Informal learning in the professions. Hull: University of Hull; 1994.

9 Grant J, Stanton F, Flood S, Mack J, Waring C. An evaluation of educational needs and provision for doctors within three years of completion of training. London: Joint Centre for Education in Medicine; 1998.

10 Todd F, ed. Planning continuing professional development. London: Croom Helm; 1987.

11 McKinley WJD. Continuing medical education 19th century style: the role of the New Sydenham Society in the education of doctors in North West England in 1866. In: Proceedings of the XXXIInd International Congress on the History of Medicine, Antwerp.

12 Beaudry JS. Effectiveness of continuing medical education: a quantitative synthesis. J Cont Educ Health Prof 1989;9:285-307.

13 Wilbur RS. Report: First International Conference on Continuing Medical Education. Rancho Mirage, California, 30 November - 4 December 1986. Med Educ 1987;21:157-64.

14 Pearson P, Jones K. Developing professional knowledge: making primary course education and research more relevant. British Medical Journal 1997;314:817–20.

15 Sackin P. Practice-based continuing medical education. Postgrad Educ Gen Pract 1990;1:2-4.

16 Allery LA, Owen PA, Robling MR. Why general practitioners and consultants change their clinical practice: a critical incident study. BMJ 1997;314:870-4.

17 Gale R, Grant J. Managing change in a medical context. Guidelines for action. London: Joint Centre for Education in Medicine; 1990.

18 Sullivan F, Mitchell E. Has general practitioner computing made a difference to patient care? A systematic review of published reports. BMJ 1995;311:848-52.

19 Feder GS, Griffthes CJ, Grimshaw JM. Healthcare practice guidelines for chronic disease management. Do they change practice? Dis Man Health Outcomes 1997;1:3129-34.

20 Nowlem PM. A new approach to continuing education for business and the professions. New York: MacMillan; 1988.

21 Abernethy RD. Continuing medical education for general practitioners in North Devon. Postgrad Med J 1990;66:847-8.

22 Stross GK. Relationships between knowledge and experience in the use of disease-modifying antirheumatic agents: a study of primary care practitioners. JAMA 1989;19:2721-3.

23 Harden RM, Laidlaw JM. Effective continuing education: The CRISIS criteria. Med Educ1992;26:408-22.

24 Conway AC, Keller RB, Wennberg DE. Partnering with physicians to achieve quality improvement. Jt Comm J Qual Improv 1995;21:619-26.

25 25 Parboosingh IJT, Thivierge RL. The Maintenance of Competence (MOCOMP) Program. Ann R Coll Phys Surg Can 1993;26:512-7.

26 Brennan B. Continuing professional education and the discipline reviews. Stud Cont Educ 1991;13:53-69.

27 Branthwaite A, Ross A, Henshaw A, Davie C. Continuing education for general practitioners: occasional paper 38. London: Royal College of General Practitioners; 1988.

28 The Royal Colleges of Physicians. Continuing medical education for the trained physician: recommendations for the introduction and implementation of a CME system. The Royal Colleges of Physicians of Edinburgh, Glasgow and London; 1994.

29 Gray DP. Continuing education for general practitioners. J R Coll Gen Pract 1988;May:195-6.

30 Moore DE. Moving CME close to the clinical encounter: the promise of quality management and CME. J Cont Educ Health Prof 1995;15:135-45.

31 Stanley I, Al-Shehri A, Thomas P. Continuing education for general practice. 1. Experience, competence and the media of self-directed learning for established general practitioners. Br J Gen Pract 1993;43:210-4.

32 Brookfield SD. Understanding and facilitating adult learning. Buckingham: Open University Press; 1986.

33 Rogers A. Learning: can we change the discourse? Adult Learn 1997;Jan:116-117.

34 Cervero RM. Effective continuing education for professionals. San Francisco: Jossey-Bass; 1988.

35 Schon D. Educating the reflective practitioner, 2nd edn. San Francisco: Jossey-Bass; 1987.

36 Stanton F, Grant J. Approaches to experiential learning in medicine. A background document. London: Joint Centre for Education in Medicine; 1998. ISBN 1873207913.

37 Houle CO. Continuing learning in the professions. San Francisco: Jossey-Bass; 1980.

38 Shirriffs G. Continuing educational requirements for general practitioners in Grampian. J R Coll Gen Pract 1989;39:190-2.

39 Durno D, Gill GM. Survey of general practitioners' views on postgraduate education in north-east Scotland. J R Coll Gen Pract 1974;24:648-54.

40 Reedy BLEC. General practitioners and postgraduate education in the northern region: occasional paper 9. The Journal of the Royal College of General Practitioners; 1979.

41 Royal College of General Practitioners. Fellowship by assessment, 2nd edn. Occasional paper 50. Exeter: The Royal College of General Practitioners; 1995.

42 Bell G. A study which explores the feasibility of establishing general practice as multi-disciplinary training practices. Sunderland Health Authority; 1996.

43 Joint Centre for Education in Medicine. Assessing and improving in general practice. Feasibility study. Confidential Report to the NHSE Development Unit. 1997.

44 UEMS. Charter on Continuing Medical Education of Medical Specialists in the European Union. Brussels: Union Européenne des Medicins Specialistes; 1994.

45 Allery L, Owen P, Hayes T, Harding K. Differences in continuing medical education activities and attitudes between trainers and trainees in general practice. Postgrad Educ Gen Pract 1991;2:176-82.

46 British Postgraduate Medical Federation. The quality of continuing medical education for general practitioners. London: British Postgraduate Medical Federation; 1993.

47 Grant J. CME. Its validation and outcome. In: Mansfield A, editor. CME and the Royal College of Surgeons. Abstracts of the 1st Conference Held at the Royal Society of Medicine: 'British Continuing Medical Education: a Framework for the Future' (4th and 5th July). 1994.

48 Fish D, Coles C. Learning through the critical appreciation of practice. Butterworth: Heinemann; 1998.

49 Harrison B. CME. A trust view. In: Mansfield A, editor. CME and the Royal College of Surgeons. Abstracts of the 1st Conference Held at the Royal Society of Medicine: 'British Continuing Medical Education: a Framework for the Future' (4th and 5th July). 1994.

50 Hollwitz J, Danielson MA. Measure the place before you measure the people: new alternatives for quality assessment. Assess Eval Higher Educ 1995;20:67-76.

51 Havener WM, Worrell P. Environmental factors in professional development activities

- does type of academic library affiliation make a difference? Lib Inf Sci Res 1994;16:318-20.

52   Kelly MH, Murray TS. Motivation of general practitioners attending postgraduate education. Br J Gen Pract 1996;46:353-6.

53   Graham I. I believe therefore I practice. Lancet 1996;347:4-5.

54   Crandall SJS, Cunliff AE. Experience with mandatory continuing education in a teaching hospital. J Cont Educ Health Prof 1989;9:155-63.

55   Walton HJ. Continuing medical education and changes in doctors. Med Educ 1991;25:1-2.

56   Jones N, Fear N. Continuing professional development - perspectives from human-resource professionals. Pers Rev 1994;23:49-60.

57   Lewis AP, Bolden KJ. General practitioners and their learning styles. J R Coll Gen Pract 1989;39:187-9.

58   Langsner SJ. Deterrents to participation in continuing professional education: a survey of the NTRS. Ther Rec J 1994;28:147-62.

59   Ferguson A. Evaluating the purpose and benefits of continuing education in nursing and the implications for the provision of continuing education for cancer nurses. J Adv Nurs 1994;19:640-6.

60   Mazmanian PE, Williams RB, Desch CE, Johnson RE. Theory and research for the development of continuing education in the health professions. J Cont Educ Health Prof 1990;10:349-65.

61   Glazier R, Buchbinder R, Bell M. Critical appraisal of continuing medical education in the rheumatic diseases for primary care physicians. Arth Rheum 1995;38:533-8.

62   Davis DA, Thomson MA, Oxmon AD, Haynes B. Evidence for the effectiveness of CME. A Review of 50 randomised control trials. JAMA 1992;268:1111-7.

63   Allan J. Learning outcomes in higher education. Stud Higher Educ 1996;21:93-108.

64   Bertram DA, Brooks-Bertram PA. The evaluation of continuing medical education: a literature review. Health Educ Mono 1977;5:330-62.

65   Jacobson LD, Edwards AE, Granier SK, Butler CC. Evidence-based medicine and general practice. Br J Gen Pract 1997;47:449-52.

66   Charlton G. Megatrials are based on a methodological mistake. Br J Gen Pract 1996;46:429-31.

67   Davidson R, Sensakovic J, Helm C, Saunders S. The effect of CME on physicians' counseling, testing, and management of HIV infection. J Cont Educ Health Prof 1990;10:303-13.

68   Davis DA. A critical analysis of the literature evaluating CME. Möbius 1987;7:87-95.

69   Dall'Alba G, Sandberg J. Educating for Competence in Professional Practice. Instr Sci 1996;24:411-37.

70   Wergin JF, Mazmanian PE, Miller WW, Papp KK, Williams WL. CME and change in practice: an alternative perspective. J Cont Educ Health Prof 1988;8:147-59.

71   Van der Vleuten CPM. The assessment of professional competence: developments, research and practical implications. Adv Health Sci Educ 1996;1:41-67.

72   Al-Shehri A, Bligh J, Stanley I. A draft charter for general practice continuing education. Postgrad Educ Gen Pract 1993;4:161-7.

73   Cividin TM, Ottoson JM. Linking reasons for continuing professional education participation with postprogram application. J Cont Educ Health Prof 1997;17:46-55.

74   Davis DA, Thomson MA, Oxman AD, Haynes B. Changing physician performance: a systematic review of the effect of continuing medical education strategies. JAMA 1995;274:700-5.

75   Fox RD, Mazmanian PE, Putnam WR. Changing and learning in the lives of physicians. New York: Praeger; 1989.

76   Jolly B, Grant J. Good assessment guide. London: Joint Centre for Education in Medicine; 1997.

77   Norman GR, van der Vleuten CPM, de Graaf E. Pitfalls in the pursuit of objectivity: issues of validity, efficiency and acceptability. Med Educ 1991;25:119-26.

78   Benett Y. The validity and reliability of assessment and self-assessments of work-based learning. Assess Eval Higher Educ 1993;18:83-94.

79   Van der Vleuten CPM, Norman GR, de Graaf E. Pitfalls in the pursuit of objectivity: issues of reliability. Med Educ 1991;25:110-8.

80   Gibbs G, Morgan A, Taylor E. The world of the learner. In: Al-Shehri *et al.* (1993),
81   1984.

      81 Boud DC. How to help students learn from experience. In: Al-Shehri *et al.* (1993),
82   1988.

      Alexander MA. Evaluation of a training program in breast cancer nursing. J Cont
83   Educ Nurs 1990;21:260-6*.

      Gerrard J, Holden JM, Elliott SA, McKenzie P, McKenzie J, Cox JL. A trainer's perspective of an innovative program teaching health visitors about the detection,
84   treatment and prevention of postnatal depression. J Adv Nurs 1993;18:1825-32*.

      Malenka DJ, O'Connor GT. A regional collaborative effort for CQI in cardiovascular disease. Northern New England Cardiovascular Study Group. Jt Comm J Qual Improv
85   1995a ;21:627-33*.

      Hadiyono JE, Suryawati S, Danu SS, Sunartono S, Santoso B. Interactional group discussion: results of a controlled trial using a behavioral intervention to reduce the
86   use of injections in public health facilities. Soc Sci Med 1996;42:1177-83*.

      Mann KV, Langille DB, Weld VP, Maccara ME, Cogdon A, Davidson K. Multidisciplinary learning in continuing professional education: The Heart Health
87   Nova Scotia experience. J Cont Educ Health Prof 1996;16:50-60*.

      Fleming RM, Fleming DM, Gaede R. Training physicians and health care providers to
88   accurately read coronary arteriograms. A training program. Angiology 1996;47:349-59*.

89   Crandall SJS. The role of continuing medical education in changing and learning. J Cont Educ Health Prof 1990;10:339–48*.

      Mansfield A, editor. CME and the Royal College of Surgeons. Abstracts of the 1st
90   Conference held at the Royal Society of Medicine: 'British Continuing Medical Education: A Framework for the Future' (4th and 5th July).

      Dalton JA, Blau W, Carlson J, Mann JD, Bernard S, Toomey T, Pierce S, Germino B. Changing the relationship among nurses' knowledge, self-reported behavior, and
91   documented behavior in pain management: does education make a difference. J Pain and Symptom Manage 1996;12:308-19 *.

92   De Buda Y, Woolf CR. Saturday at the University: a format for success. J Cont Educ Health Prof 1990;10:279-84*.

93   Parboosingh IJT. Learning portfolios: potential to assist health professionals with self directed learning. J Cont Educ Health Prof 1996;16:75-81.

      Davis D, Thomson MA. Implications for undergraduate and graduate education
94   derived from quantitative research in continuing medical education: lessons learned from an automobile. J Cont Educ Health Prof 1996;16:159-66.

      Williamson JW, German PS, Weiss R, Skinner EA, Bowes FIII. Health science
95   information management and continuing education of physicians: a survey of US primary care practitioners and their opinion leaders. Ann Int Med 1989;110:151-60.

96   Dunn WR, Hamilton DD. Competence-based education and distance learning: a tandem for professional continuing education. Stud Higher Educ 1985;10:277-87.

97   Tracey JM, Arroll B, Richmond DE, Barnham PM. The validity of general practitioners' self-assessment of knowledge: cross sectional study. BMJ 1997;315:1426-8.

      Wiles R. Quality questions. Nursing Times 1996;October 30, Vol. 92, No 44:38-40.

98   Chambers E, Grant J, Jackson G. The good CME guide. London: Joint Centre for Education in Medicine; 1998.

99   Green L, Kreuter M, Deeds S, Partridge K. Health education planning: a diagnostic approach. Palo Alto, CA: Mayfield Press; 1980.

100   Green LW, Kreuter MW. Health promotion planning: an educational and environmental approach. Palo Alto, CA: Mayfield Press; 1991.

101   Davis MH, Harden RM, Laidlaw JM, Pitts NB, Paterson RD, Watts A, Saunders WP. Continuing education for general dental practitioners using a printed distance learning programme. Med Educ 1992;26:378–83.

102 Ottoson JM. Use of a conceptual framework to explore multiple influences on the application of learning following a continuing education program. Can J Stud Adult
103 Learn 1995;9:1-18.
Grilli R, Lomas J. Evaluating the message: The relationship between compliance rate and subject of a practice guideline. Med Care 1994;32:202-13.

FURTHER READING

Abbott L et al. Videoconferencing in Continuing Education: an evaluation of its application to professional development at the University of Ulster (1990-95). Educ Media Int 1995;32:77-82.

Amesberger G. Evaluation of experiential learning programmes: qualitative and quantitative approaches. J Advent Educ Outdoor Leadership 1996;13:58-62.

Bachman JA, Kitchens EK, Halley SS, Ellison KJ. Assessment of learning needs of nurse educators: continuing education implications. J Cont Educ Nurs 1992;23:29-33.

Becher T. The learning professions. Stud Higher Educ 1996;21:43-55.

Bellack JP. Characteristics and outcomes of a statewide nurse refresher project. J Cont Educ Nurs 1995;26:60-6.

Bennett NL, Casebeer LL. Evolution of planning in CME. J Cont Educ Health Prof 1995;15:70-9.

Biddle C. AANA journal course: update for nurse anesthetists – outcome measures in anesthesiology: are we going in the right direction? AANA J 1994;62:117-24.

Blanchard D, Fox RD. A profile of nonurban physicians from the study of changing and learning in the lives of physicians. J Cont Educ Health Prof 1990;10:329-38.

Brady L. Assessing curriculum outcomes in australian schools. Educ Rev 1997;49:57-65.

Burge EJ et al. The Audioconference: delivering continuing education for addictions workers in Canada. J Alc Drug Educ 1993;39:78-91.

Burrows P. Continuing medical education and pharmaceutical sponsorship. Postgrad Educ Gen Pract 1990;1:115-6.

Campbell C, Gondocz T, Parboosingh IJT. Documenting and managing self-directed learning among specialists. Ann R Coll of Phys Surg Can 1995;28:80-4.

Cantwell ZM. School-based leadership and professional socialization of the assistant principal. Urban Educ 1993;28:49-68.

Carr A. Clinical psychology in Ireland - a national survey. Irish J Psychol 1995;16:1-20.

Cervero RM. The importance of practical knowledge and implications for continuing education. J Cont Educ Health Prof 1990;10:85-94.

Cervero RM, Rottet S. Analyzing the effectiveness of continuing professional education: an exploratory study. Adult Educ Quart 1984;34:135-46.

Challis M, Mathers NJ, Howe AC, Field NJ. Portfolio-based learning: continuing medical education for general practitioners - a mid-point evaluation. Med Educ 1997;31:22-6.

Cornell JM, Kahn EH, Bahrawy AA. The School Nurse Development Program: an experiment in off-site delivery. J Cont Educ Nurs 1992;23:127-33*.

D'Alessandro MP, Galvin JR, Erkonen WE, Curry DS, Flanagan JR, D'Alessandro DM, Lacey DL, Wagner JR. The Virtual Hospital: an IAIMS continuing education into the work flow.

MD Comput 1996;13:323-9.

Department of Health and the Welsh Office. General practice in the national health service: a new contract. London: HMSO; 1989.

Department of Health. Primary care: choice and opportunity. London: HMSO 1996a.

Department of Health. Primary care: delivering the future. London: HMSO 1996b.

Department of Health. The National Health Service: a service with ambitions. London: HMSO 1996c.

Docking S. Professional development through distance learning: the professional nurses accredited learning scheme. Prof Nurs 1993;9:38-41.

Ebel R. The practical validation of tests of ability. Educ Measure: Issues Pract 1983;2:7-10.

Emens JM. Intractible vaginal discharge. PACE review for the Royal College of Obstetricians and Gynaecologists. 1995.

Falvo DR. Educational evaluation: what are the outcomes? Adv Renal Replace Ther 1995;2:227-33.

Feest T. NVQs in publishing, - why bother? Learned Publ 1996;9:79-85.

Fox RD. New horizons for research in continuing medical education. Acad Med 1990;65:550-5.

Glazier RH, Dalby DM, Badley EM, Hawker GA, Bell MJ, Buchbinder R. Determinants of physician confidence in the primary care management of musculoskeletal disorders. J Rheumatol 1996;23:351-6.

Goodsman D. Continuing professional development. London: Joint Centre for Education in Medicine; 1994.

Gottfried SS, Kyle WC. Textbook use and the biology education desired state. J Res Sci Teach 1992;29:35–49.

Grotelveschen AD, Hamish DL, Kenny WR. An analysis of the participation reasons scale administered to business professionals. Occasional paper 7. Urbana: Office for the Study of Continuing Professional Education, University of Illinois at Urbana-Champaign; 1979.

Hager P, Gonczi A, Athanasou J. General issues about assessment of competence. Assess Eval Higher Educ 1994;19:3-16.

Harmes HM, Sullivan DE. A study of long-term outcomes of return-to-industry programs. Comm Coll Rev 1994;22:48-54.

Headrick L, Katcher W, Neuhauser D, McEachern E. Continuous quality improvement and knowledge for improvement applied to asthma care. Jt Comm J Qual Improv 1994;20:562-8.

Hedman L, Lazure LA. Extending continuing education to rural area nurses. J Cont Educ Nurs 1990;21:165-8.

Helsby G. Defining and developing professionalism in english secondary-schools. J Educ

Teach 1996;22:135-48.

Hoftvedt BO, Mjell J. Referrals: peer review as continuing medical education. Teach Learn Med 1993;5:234-7.

Hoftvedt BO, Paus A, Natrud E, Sandsmark M, Schøyen R, Sundelin F. Evaluating a management training program for hospital doctors in Norway. J Cont Educ Health Prof 1995;15:91-4.

Hughes RB, Cummings H, Allen RV. The Nurse Extern Practicum: a new partnership between education and service. J Nurs Staff Develop 1993;9:118-21.

Iphofen R, Poland F. Professional empowerment and teaching sociology to health care professionals. Teaching Sociology 1997;25:44-56.

Jackson BJ, Hays BJ, Robinson CC. Multiple delivery methods for an interdisciplinary audience: assessing effectiveness. J Cont Educ Health Prof 1990;10:59-69.

Jacobsen C, Malan S, Perkins T, Slatten R. A regional approach to entry-level critical care education. Focus Crit Care 1990;17:385-6*.

Jansen JJM, Scherpbier AJJA, Metz JCM, Grol RPTM, van der Vleuten CPM, Rethans JJ. Performance-based assessment in continuing medical education for general practitioners: construct validity. Med Educ 1996;30:339-44.

Jansen JJM, Tan LHC, van der Vleuten CPM, van Linjk SJ, Rethans JJ, Grol RPTM. Assessment of competence in technical clinical skills of general practitioners. Med Educ 1995;25:414-20.

Järvinin A, Konoven V. Promoting professional development in higher education through portfolio assessment. Assess Eval Higher Educ 1995;20:25-36.

Jasper MA. The potential of the professional portfolio for nursing. J Clin Nurs 1995;4:249-55.

Jennett PA, Laxdal OE, Hayton RC, Klaasen DJ, Swanson RW, Wilson TS, Spooner HJ, Mainprize GW, Wicket REY. The effects of continuing medical education on family doctor performance in office practice: a randomised control study. Med Educ 1988;22:139-45.

Jennett PA, Scott SM, Atkinson MA, Crutcher RA, Hogan DB, Elford RW, Maccannell KL, Baumber JS. Patients charts and physician office management decisions: chart audit and chart stimulated recall. J Cont Educ Health Prof 1995;15:31-9.

Johns C, Graham J. The growth of management connoisseurship through reflective practice. J Nurs Manage 1994;2:253-60.

Kalnins I, Phelps SL, Glauber W. Outcomes of nurse (RN) refresher courses in a midwestern city. J Cont Educ Nurs 1994;25:268-71.

Kelly MH, Murray TS. Who are the providers of medical education? Med Educ 1993;27:452-60.

Madlon-Kay DJ. Improvement in family physician recognition and treatment of hypercholesterolemia. Arch Int Med 1989;149:1754-5.

Loughridge B, Oates J, Speight S. Career development - follow-up studies of Sheffield MA graduates 1985/1986-92/1993. J Lib and Inf Sci 1996;28:105-17.

Lexchin J. Interactions between physicians and the pharmaceutical industry: what does the literature say? Can Med Assoc J 1993;149:1401-7.

Langham S, Gillam S, Thorogood M. The carrot, the stick, and the general practitioner: how have changes in financial incentives affected health promotion in general practice? Br J Gen Pract 1995;45:665-8.

Lane DS. Outcome measurement in multi-interventional continuing medical education. J Cont Educ Health Prof 1997;17:12-9*.

Kuramoto AM, Wyman JA. Design and implementation of effective delivery approaches for continuing nursing education. Möbius 1986;6:6-10.

Kopp ME, Schell KA, Laskowski-Jones L, Morelli PK. Critical care nurse internships: in theory and practice. Crit Care Nurs 1993;13:115-8.

Knox AB. Influences on participation in continuing education. J Cont Educ Health Prof 1990;19:261-74.

Knowles MS. Self-directed learning: a guide for learners and teachers. Cambridge: Cambridge Books; 1975.

Klayman J, Brown K. Debias the environment instead of the judge: an alternative approach to reducing error in diagnostic (and other) judgment. Cognition 1993;49:97-122*.

Kerr DNS. The value of CME. In: Abstracts of the Second Conference Held at the Royal Society in Medicine: 'British Continuing Medical Educ: a Framework for the Future' (15th and 16th Sept). 1994.

Mayne K. Practice-linked continuing medical education. Med J Aust 1994;161:630-2.

McAuley RG, Paul WM, Morrison GH, Beckett RF, Goldsmith CH. Five year results of the peer assessment program of the College of Physicians and Surgeons of Ontario. Can Med Assoc J 1990;143:1193-9.

McClennan BL, Herlihy CS. The continuing competence needs of physicians: a survey of the medical specialty societies. Am J Roentgenol 1995;165:789-95.

McGuire C. The curriculum for the year 2000. Med Educ 1989;23:221-7 1990.

McKnight A, Bradley T. How do general practitioners qualify for their PGEA? Br J Gen Pract 1996;46:679-80.

Melton R. Learning outcomes for higher education: some key issues. Br J Educ Stud 1996;44:409-25.

Millar C. Educating the educators of adults: two cheers for curriculum negotiation. J Curric Stud 1989;21:161-8.

Moore P, Pace KB, Rapacz K. Collaborative model for continuing education for home health nurses. J Cont Educ Nurs 1991;22:67-72.

Morrow NC, Hargie ODW. Influencing and persuading skills at the interprofessional interface: training for action. J Cont Educ Health Prof 1996;16:94-102.

Murdock JE, Neafsey PJ. Self-efficacy measurements: an approach for predicting practice outcomes in continuing education? J Cont Educ Nurs 1995;26:158-65.

Murray TS, Dyker GS, Campbell LM. Characteristics of general practitioners who are high attenders at educational meetings. Br J Gen Pract 1992a;42:157-9.

Murray TS, Dyker GS, Campbell LM. Continuing medical education and the education allowance: variation in credits obtained by GPs. Med Educ 1992b;26:248-50.

Murray TS, Dyker GS, Campbell LM. Postgraduate education allowance: general practitioners' attendance at courses outwith their region. Br J Gen Pract 1992c;42:194-6.

Okey A et al. Surveying the effectiveness of short course-provision in the professional development of library and information specialists. J Educ Lib Inf Sc 1992;33:249-53.

Paget NS, Saunders NA, Newble NA, Du J. Physician assessment pilot study for the Royal Australasian College of Physicians. J Cont Educ Health Prof 1996;16:103-11.

Parboosingh IJT, Campbell CM, Gondocz T. Development of a standard for self-directed continuing medical education. Ann R Coll Phys Surg Can 1995;28:75-8.

Parboosingh IJT, Gondocz ST, Lai A. The annual MOCOMP profile. Ann R Coll Phys Surg Can 1993;26:544-7

Parker DJ, Gray HH, Balcon R, Birkhead JS, Boyle RM, Hutton I, Parsons L, Rothman MT, Shaw TR. Planning for coronary angioplasty: guidelines for training and continuing competence. British Cardiac Society (BCS) and British Cardiovascular Intervention Society (BCIS) working group on interventional cardiology. Heart 1996;75:419-25.

Pickup AJ, Mee LG, Hedley AJ. The general practitioner and continuing education. Br J Gen Pract 1983;33:486-92.

Pinion SB. Conservative alternatives to hysterectomy for dysfunctional uterine bleeding. PACE review for the Royal College of Obstetricians and Gynaecologists. 1994.

Piterman L. GPs as learners. Med J Aust 1991;155:318-22.

Pories WJ, Smout JC, Morris A, Lewkow VE. U.S. Health care reform: will it change postgraduate surgical education? World J Surg 1994;18:745-52.

Purnell L. Outcomes of a university-based registered nurse refresher course: a 5-year follow-up. J Nurs Staff Develop 1995;11:31-4.

Ramsden P. Improving learning: new perspectives. London: Kogan Page; 1988.

Raymond M. Continuing education in the health professions: a reanalysis of the literature. Paper presented at the meeting of the American Educational Research Association, San Francisco. 1986.

Robb AJP, Murray R. Medical humanities in nursing - thought provoking. J Adv Nurs 1992;17:1182-7.

Rogers EM. Diffusion of innovations. New York: Free Press; 1983.

Rolfe IE, Andrei JM, Pearson S, Hensley MS, Gordon JJ. Clinical competence of interns. Med Educ 1995;29:225-30.

Royal Society of Medicine. Yearbook of Continuing Medical Education. London: The Royal Society of Medicine Press 1995.

Sachdeva AK. Preceptorship, mentorship, and the adult learner in medical and health sciences education. J Canc Educ 1996;11:131-6.

Sandmire HF, DeMott RK. The Green Bay Cesarean Section Study. III. Falling cesarean birth rates without a formal curtailment program. Am J Obstetric Gynecolog 1994;170:1790-9.

Saul JL. Action outcome evaluation: a case study. J Cont Higher Educ 1992;40:18-21*.

Saywell RM, Jay SJ, Lukas PJ, Casebeer LL, Mybeck KC, Parchman ML, Haley AJ. Indiana family physician attitudes and practices concerning smoking cessation. Indiana Med 1996;89:149-56.

Scheller MK. A qualitative analysis of factors in the work environment that influence nurses' use of knowledge gained from CE programs. J Cont Educ Nurs 1993;24:114-22.

SCMCDCME. Future Directions for Medical College Continuing Medical Education. Washington: Society of Medical Directors of CME; 1995.

Seitz JA. A collaborative approach to professional development. J Cont Higher Educ 1995;43:44-53.

Shenk D, Lee J. Meeting the educational needs of service providers: effects of a continuing education program on self-reported knowledge and attitudes about aging. Educ Gerontol 1995;21:671-81*.

Sibley JC, Sackett DL, Neufeld V, Gerrard B, Rudnick KV, Fraser W. A randomised control trial of continuing medical education. NEJM 1982;306:511-5.

Stokes RA. Streamlining orientation for haemodialysis nursing: a competency-based approach. ANNA J 1991;18:33-8.

Swedish Medical Association. Continuing medical education in sweden: an educational policy program. Stockholm: Swedish Medical Association; 1995.

Tjeltveit AC. The psychotherapist as Christian ethicist – theology applied to practice. J Psychol Theol 1992;20:89-98.
Tolnai S. Continuing medical education and career choice among graduates of problem-based and traditional curricula. Med Educ 1991;25:414-20.

Van Harrison R, Gallay LS, McKay NE, Calhoun JG, Calhoun GL, Oh MS. The association between community physicians' attendance at a medical center's CME courses and their patient referrals to the medical centre. J Cont Educ Health Prof 1990;10:315-20.

Vickrey BG. Outcomes research - possible effects on clinical practice. West J Med 1993;159:183-4.

Volberding PA. Improving the outcomes of care for patients with Human Immunodeficiency Virus infection. NEJM 1996;334:729-31.

Walsh JME, McPhee SJ. A systems model for clinical preventive care: an analysis of factors influence patient and physician. Health Educ Quart 1992;19:157-75.

Walton HJ. Continuing medical education in Europe: a survey. Med Educ 1994;28:333-42.

Weerakoon PK, Fernando DN. Self-evaluation of skills as a method of assessing learning needs for continuing education. Med Teach 1991;13:103-6.

Williams AR, Davis RD, Hale CD, Collins TR. Patterns of concern: needs assessment and continuing education needs among public health physicians. J Cont Educ Health Prof 1989;9:131-9.

Young Y, Brigley S, Littlejohns P, McEwen J. Continuing education for public health medicine - is it just another paper exercise? J Publ Health Med 1996;18:357-63.

Woolf CR. Personal continuing education relationships between perceived needs by individual physicians and practice profiles. J Cont Educ Health Prof 1988;8:271-6.